My Little Helper

A Personal Medical History

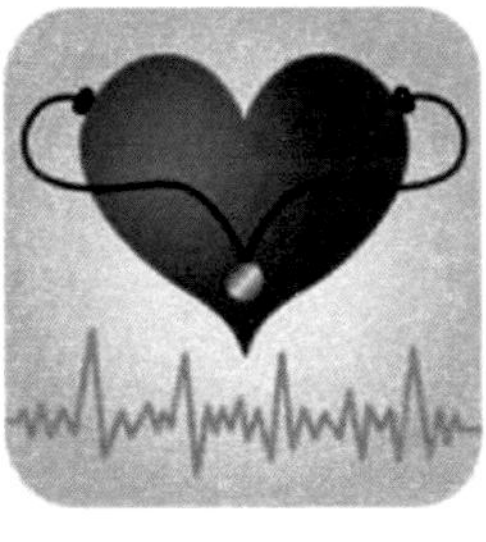

Nicole Davis

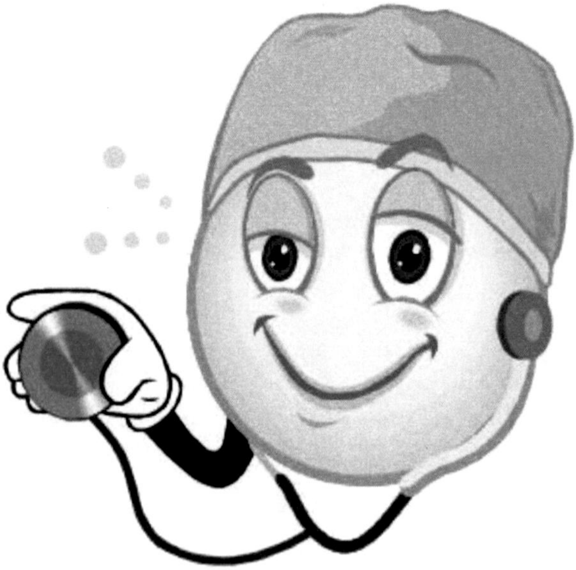

Patients Name

Nombre de los pacientes

Diagnosis

Diagnóstico

Date Record Started

Fecha de Registro de inicio

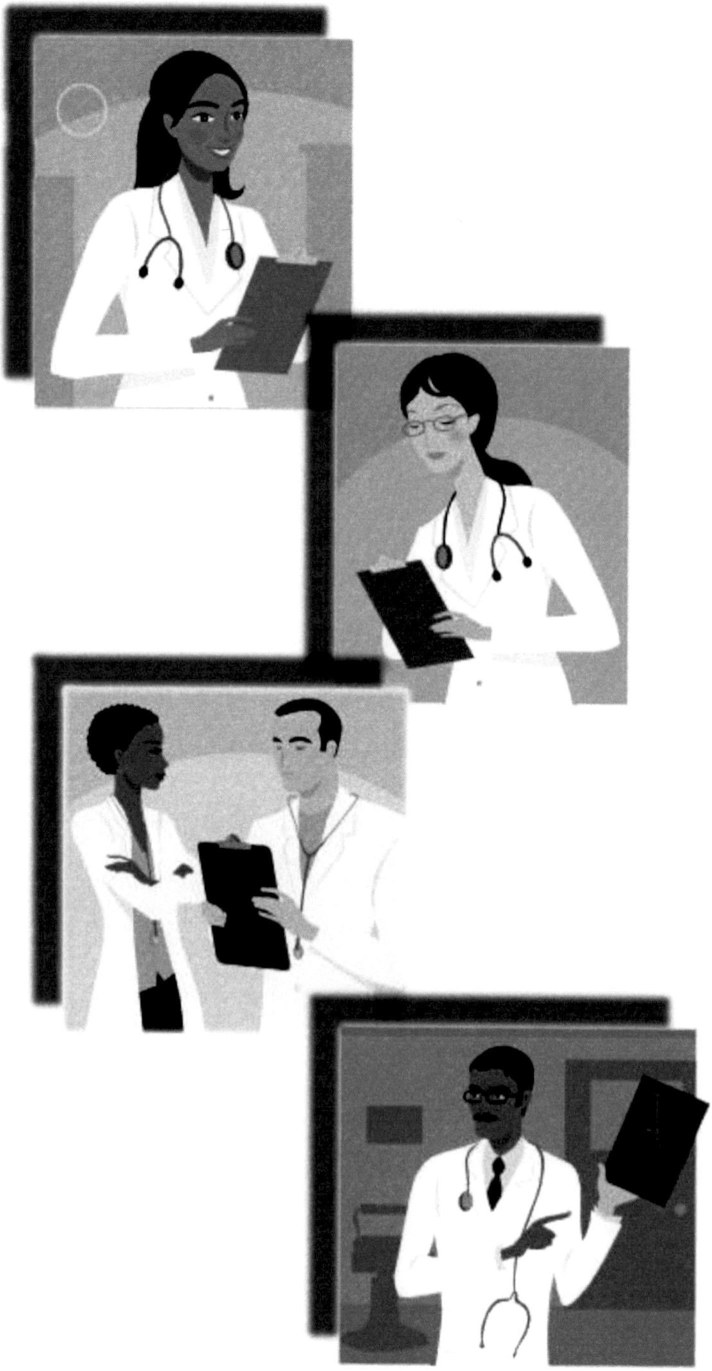

If found, please return this book to:

Si se encuentra, por favor devuelva este libro a:

ISBN 0-9777235-2-6
978-0-9777235-2-2

First Edition, June 2009
Printed in the United States of America
Writers Cramp Publishing
http://www.writerscramp.us

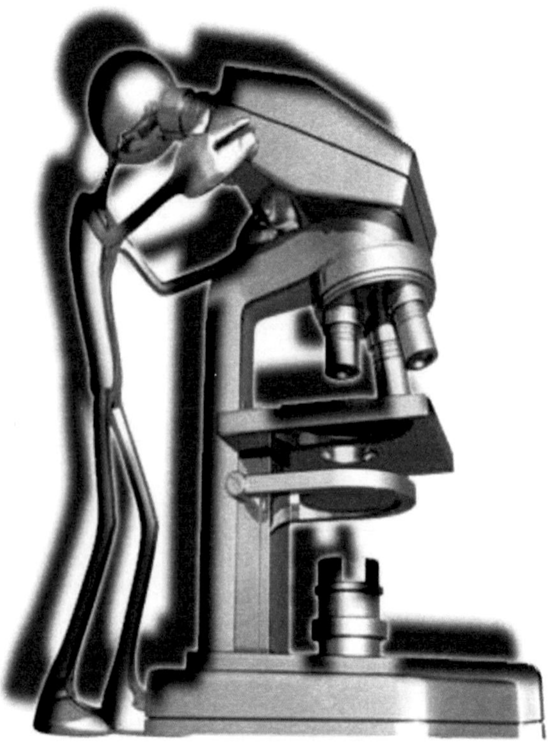

Table of Contents

SUMMARY **1**
Resumen

DOCTORS / HEALTH PROFESSIONALS **5**
Médicos / Profesionales de la Salud

ALLERGIES **15**
Alergias

MEDICATIONS **19**
Medicamentos

SCANS, X-RAYS, TESTS, ETC **27**
Exploraciones, rayos X, pruebas, etc

SURGERIES **37**
Cirugías

TRANSFUSIONS **43**
Transfusiones

CHEMOTHERAPY **47**
Quimioterapia

TRANSPLANTS **53**
Trasplantes

OTHER PROCEDURES **55**
Otros Procedimientos

TEMPERATURE **63**
Temperatura

NOTES/PHONE NUMBERS **69**
Notas / Numeros de Teléfono

APPENDIX A: MONTHLY CALENDARS **77**

APPENDIX B: GENERAL CHART **89**

APPENDIX C: WEEKLY SUGAR GRAPH **91**

APPENDIX D: SIX MONTHS CHART **93**

APPENDIX E: LIST OF WEBSITES **95**

My Little Helper is designed to be a convenient summary of an individual's medical history over a lifetime, or a place to record the pertinent details as you or your loved one goes through a serious illness or injury. Designed using spiral binding, it is intended to be laid flat and copied. This is an invaluable reference when filling out paperwork for a new doctor, bringing the night nurse up to speed, or worse, that midnight trip to the emergency room.

It's during the most trying times that the value of this reference is most apparent. Documented properly and kept up to date, ***My Little Helper*** can alleviate stress and frustration when you're relating what happened months or even years before.

Summary: Use this area to maintain a quick medical history of the individual. For example: leukemia first detected June 2008; deathly allergic to penicillin; etc. Keep it neat and simple. In the event of an emergency, and the doctors or EMTs need to know the details of your condition fast, all the critical information is here. Print because it's important that they can easily read what you write.

Doctors: List all the doctors and relevant health professionals that you have seen. Make sure to include your primary care provider and any specialists including anesthesiologists, chiropractor, dentists, oral surgeons, etc.

Allergies: List all allergies you have. Make sure to be specific here. Don't just put down medications but include things like foods, adhesives, latex, etc.

Medications: List all medications that you have taken both past and present. The first listing on each page has more space for any dosage changes that may occur over time.

Surgeries: Write an overview of the procedure and include any reactions, issues, etc. Include surgeons, anesthesiologists and even those consulted as a second opinion. Don't be afraid of putting data in more than one place in your book.

Scans, X-rays, Tests, etc: Keep track of MRI's, X-rays, bone scans, blood tests, urine tests, etc.

Transfusions: List all transfusions. Include reactions and any problems.

Chemotherapy: List all chemotherapies. Include reactions and how you are feeling emotionally and physically.

Transplants: List any transplants here. (kidney, bone marrow, lung, etc.)

Other Procedures: Any other general procedures you wish to record. (i.e. wisdom teeth removed)

Temperature: Most medical institutions and those who work within them prefer to talk about temperature in Celsius. For those who think in Fahrenheit, here are two easy ways to convert. Use the extended tables to track fever during critical times to help the doctors evaluate patterns.

Notes/Phone Numbers: Use this as a notepad to keep track of those little reminders or as your medical phone book. It never hurts to have a phone number in more than one place in this book.

Buy a three-ring binder and put copies of the Appendix's in it or use them as-is in your book.

Appendix A: Monthly Calendars: Use the monthly calendars to keep track of those important appointments.

Appendix B: General Chart: Fill in the column headers to create your own charts for your specific needs.

Appendix C: Two Week Blood Sugar Graph: Mark with a colored dot to graph twice daily sugar levels over two weeks.

Appendix D: Six Months Chart: A general log of twice daily data over six months. Use for sugar levels, blood pressure, etc.

Appendix E: List of Websites: Some of the major websites where medical information and help can be found.

Summary

Summary

Doctors / Health Professionals

Name/*Nombre*

Phone/ *Teléfono*

Address/ *Dirección*

Specialty/ *Especialidad*

Name

Phone

Address

Specialty

Name

Phone

Address

Specialty

Name

Phone

Address

Specialty

Name

Phone

Address

Specialty

Name

Phone

Address

Specialty

Médicos / Profesionales de la Salud

Name/*Nombre*

Phone/*Teléfono*

Address/ *Dirección*

Specialty/ *Especialidad*

Name

Phone

Address

Specialty

Name

Phone

Address

Specialty

Name

Phone

Address

Specialty

Name

Phone

Address

Specialty

Name

Phone

Address

Specialty

Doctors / Health Professionals

Name/*Nombre*

Phone/*Teléfono*

Address/ *Dirección*

Specialty/ *Especialidad*

Name

Phone

Address

Specialty

Name

Phone

Address

Specialty

Name

Phone

Address

Specialty

Name

Phone

Address

Specialty

Name

Phone

Address

Specialty

Médicos / Profesionales de la Salud

Name/*Nombre*

Phone/*Teléfono*

Address/ *Dirección*

Specialty/ *Especialidad*

Name

Phone

Address

Specialty

Name

Phone

Address

Specialty

Name

Phone

Address

Specialty

Name

Phone

Address

Specialty

Name

Phone

Address

Specialty

Doctors / Health Professionals

Name/*Nombre*

Phone/*Teléfono*

Address/ *Dirección*

Specialty/ *Especialidad*

Name

Phone

Address

Specialty

Name

Phone

Address

Specialty

Name

Phone

Address

Specialty

Name

Phone

Address

Specialty

Name

Phone

Address

Specialty

Médicos / Profesionales de la Salud

Name/*Nombre*

Phone/*Teléfono*

Address/ *Dirección*

Specialty/ *Especialidad*

Name

Phone

Address

Specialty

Name

Phone

Address

Specialty

Name

Phone

Address

Specialty

Name

Phone

Address

Specialty

Name

Phone

Address

Specialty

Doctors / Health Professionals

Name/*Nombre*

Phone/*Teléfono*

Address/ *Dirección*

Specialty/ *Especialidad*

Name

Phone

Address

Specialty

Name

Phone

Address

Specialty

Name

Phone

Address

Specialty

Name

Phone

Address

Specialty

Name

Phone

Address

Specialty

Médicos / Profesionales de la Salud

Name/*Nombre*

Phone/*Teléfono*

Address/ *Dirección*

Specialty/ *Especialidad*

Name

Phone

Address

Specialty

Name

Phone

Address

Specialty

Name

Phone

Address

Specialty

Name

Phone

Address

Specialty

Name

Phone

Address

Specialty

Doctors / Health Professionals

Name/*Nombre*

Phone/*Teléfono*

Address/ *Dirección*

Specialty/ *Especialidad*

Name

Phone

Address

Specialty

Name

Phone

Address

Specialty

Name

Phone

Address

Specialty

Name

Phone

Address

Specialty

Name

Phone

Address

Specialty

Médicos / Profesionales de la Salud

Name/*Nombre*

Phone/*Teléfono*

Address/ *Dirección*

Specialty/ *Especialidad*

Name

Phone

Address

Specialty

Name

Phone

Address

Specialty

Name

Phone

Address

Specialty

Name

Phone

Address

Specialty

Name

Phone

Address

Specialty

Allergies

Name / *Nombre*

Reaction / *Reacción*

Treatment / *Tratamiento*

Name

Reaction

Treatment

Name

Reaction

Treatment

Name

Reaction

Treatment

Name

Reaction

Treatment

Name

Reaction

Treatment

Name

Reaction

Treatment

Name

Reaction

Treatment

Name

Reaction

Treatment

Name / *Nombre*
Reaction / *Reacción*
Treatment / *Tratamiento*
Name
Reaction
Treatment
Name
Reaction
Treatment
Name
Reaction
Treatment
Name
Reaction
Treatment
Name
Reaction
Treatment
Name
Reaction
Treatment
Name
Reaction
Treatment
Name
Reaction
Treatment

Allergies

Name / *Nombre*

Reaction / *Reacción*

Treatment / *Tratamiento*

Name

Reaction

Treatment

Name

Reaction

Treatment

Name

Reaction

Treatment

Name

Reaction

Treatment

Name

Reaction

Treatment

Name

Reaction

Treatment

Name

Reaction

Treatment

Name

Reaction

Treatment

Name / *Nombre*

Reaction / *Reacción*

Treatment / *Tratamiento*

Name

Reaction

Treatment

Name

Reaction

Treatment

Name

Reaction

Treatment

Name

Reaction

Treatment

Name

Reaction

Treatment

Name

Reaction

Treatment

Name

Reaction

Treatment

Name

Reaction

Treatment

Medications

Name / *Nombre*		
What for / *Para qué*		
Dosage / *Dosis*	When / *Cuándo*	Date / *Fecha*

Name		
What for		
Dosage	How often	Date

Name		
What for		
Dosage	How often	Date

Name		
What for		
Dosage	How often	Date

Name		
What for		
Dosage	How often	Date

Name		
What for		
Dosage	How often	Date

Medicamentos

Name / *Nombre*		
What for / *Para qué*		
Dosage / *Dosis*	When / *Cuándo*	Date / *Fecha*

Name		
What for		
Dosage	How often	Date

Name		
What for		
Dosage	How often	Date

Name		
What for		
Dosage	How often	Date

Name		
What for		
Dosage	How often	Date

Name		
What for		
Dosage	How often	Date

Medications

Name / *Nombre*		
What for / *Para qué*		
Dosage / *Dosis*	When / *Cuándo*	Date / *Fecha*

Name		
What for		
Dosage	How often	Date

Name		
What for		
Dosage	How often	Date

Name		
What for		
Dosage	How often	Date

Name		
What for		
Dosage	How often	Date

Name		
What for		
Dosage	How often	Date

Medicamentos

Name / *Nombre*

What for / *Para qué*

Dosage / *Dosis*	When / *Cuándo*	Date / *Fecha*

Name

What for

Dosage	How often	Date

Name

What for

Dosage	How often	Date

Name

What for

Dosage	How often	Date

Name

What for

Dosage	How often	Date

Name

What for

Dosage	How often	Date

Medications

Name / *Nombre*		
What for / *Para qué*		
Dosage / *Dosis*	When / *Cuándo*	Date / *Fecha*

Name		
What for		
Dosage	How often	Date

Name		
What for		
Dosage	How often	Date

Name		
What for		
Dosage	How often	Date

Name		
What for		
Dosage	How often	Date

Name		
What for		
Dosage	How often	Date

Name / *Nombre*		
What for / *Para qué*		
Dosage / *Dosis*	When / *Cuándo*	Date / *Fecha*
Name		
What for		
Dosage	How often	Date
Name		
What for		
Dosage	How often	Date
Name		
What for		
Dosage	How often	Date
Name		
What for		
Dosage	How often	Date
Name		
What for		
Dosage	How often	Date

Medications

Name / *Nombre*

What for / *Para qué*

Dosage / *Dosis*	When / *Cuándo*	Date / *Fecha*

Name

What for

Dosage	How often	Date

Name

What for

Dosage	How often	Date

Name

What for

Dosage	How often	Date

Name

What for

Dosage	How often	Date

Name

What for

Dosage	How often	Date

Medicamentos

Name / *Nombre*		
What for / *Para qué*		
Dosage / *Dosis*	When / *Cuándo*	Date / *Fecha*
Name		
What for		
Dosage	How often	Date
Name		
What for		
Dosage	How often	Date
Name		
What for		
Dosage	How often	Date
Name		
What for		
Dosage	How often	Date
Name		
What for		
Dosage	How often	Date

Scans, X-Rays, Tests, etc

Type / *Tipo*	Date / *Fecha*
Location / *Lugar*	
Results / *Resultados*	

Type	Date
Location	
Results	

Type	Date
Location	
Results	

Type	Date
Location	
Results	

Type	Date
Location	
Results	

Type	Date
Location	
Results	

Exploraciones, rayos X, pruebas, etc

Type / *Tipo*	Date / *Fecha*
Location / *Lugar*	
Results / *Resultados*	

Type	Date
Location	
Results	

Type	Date
Location	
Results	

Type	Date
Location	
Results	

Type	Date
Location	
Results	

Type	Date
Location	
Results	

Scans, X-Rays, Tests, etc

Type / *Tipo*	Date / *Fecha*

Location / *Lugar*

Results / *Resultados*

Type	Date

Location

Results

Type	Date

Location

Results

Type	Date

Location

Results

Type	Date

Location

Results

Type	Date

Location

Results

Exploraciones, rayos X, pruebas, etc

Type / *Tipo*	Date / *Fecha*
Location / *Lugar*	
Results / *Resultados*	

Type	Date
Location	
Results	

Type	Date
Location	
Results	

Type	Date
Location	
Results	

Type	Date
Location	
Results	

Type	Date
Location	
Results	

Scans, X-Rays, Tests, etc

Type / *Tipo*	Date / *Fecha*
Location / *Lugar*	
Results / *Resultados*	

Type	Date
Location	
Results	

Type	Date
Location	
Results	

Type	Date
Location	
Results	

Type	Date
Location	
Results	

Type	Date
Location	
Results	

Exploraciones, rayos X, pruebas, etc

Type / *Tipo*	Date / *Fecha*
Location / *Lugar*	
Results / *Resultados*	

Type	Date
Location	
Results	

Type	Date
Location	
Results	

Type	Date
Location	
Results	

Type	Date
Location	
Results	

Type	Date
Location	
Results	

Scans, X-Rays, Tests, etc

Type / *Tipo*	Date / *Fecha*
Location / *Lugar*	
Results / *Resultados*	

Type	Date
Location	
Results	

Type	Date
Location	
Results	

Type	Date
Location	
Results	

Type	Date
Location	
Results	

Type	Date
Location	
Results	

Exploraciones, rayos X, pruebas, etc

Type / *Tipo*	Date / *Fecha*
Location / *Lugar*	
Results / *Resultados*	

Type	Date
Location	
Results	

Type	Date
Location	
Results	

Type	Date
Location	
Results	

Type	Date
Location	
Results	

Type	Date
Location	
Results	

Scans, X-Rays, Tests, etc

Type / *Tipo*	Date / *Fecha*
Location / *Lugar*	
Results / *Resultados*	

Type	Date
Location	
Results	

Type	Date
Location	
Results	

Type	Date
Location	
Results	

Type	Date
Location	
Results	

Type	Date
Location	
Results	

Exploraciones, rayos X, pruebas, etc

Type / *Tipo*	Date / *Fecha*
Location / *Lugar*	
Results / *Resultados*	

Type	Date
Location	
Results	

Type	Date
Location	
Results	

Type	Date
Location	
Results	

Type	Date
Location	
Results	

Type	Date
Location	
Results	

Surgeries

Name / *Nombre*

Date / *Fecha*

Doctor(s) / *Médico(s)*

Anesthesiologist / *Anestesiólogo*

Hospital

Notes / *Notas*

Name

Date

Doctor(s)

Anesthesiologist

Hospital

Notes

Name

Date

Doctor(s)

Anesthesiologist

Hospital

Notes

Name

Date

Doctor(s)

Anesthesiologist

Hospital

Notes

Name / *Nombre*

Date / *Fecha*

Doctor(s) / *Médico(s)*

Anesthesiologist / *Anestesiólogo*

Hospital

Notes / *Notas*

Name

Date

Doctor(s)

Anesthesiologist

Hospital

Notes

Name

Date

Doctor(s)

Anesthesiologist

Hospital

Notes

Name

Date

Doctor(s)

Anesthesiologist

Hospital

Notes

Surgeries

Name / *Nombre*

Date / *Fecha*

Doctor(s) / *Médico(s)*

Anesthesiologist / *Anestesiólogo*

Hospital

Notes / *Notas*

Name

Date

Doctor(s)

Anesthesiologist

Hospital

Notes

Name

Date

Doctor(s)

Anesthesiologist

Hospital

Notes

Name

Date

Doctor(s)

Anesthesiologist

Hospital

Notes

Name / *Nombre*

Date / *Fecha*

Doctor(s) / *Médico(s)*

Anesthesiologist / *Anestesiólogo*

Hospital

Notes / *Notas*

Name

Date

Doctor(s)

Anesthesiologist

Hospital

Notes

Name

Date

Doctor(s)

Anesthesiologist

Hospital

Notes

Name

Date

Doctor(s)

Anesthesiologist

Hospital

Notes

Surgeries

Name / *Nombre*

Date / *Fecha*

Doctor(s) / *Médico(s)*

Anesthesiologist / *Anestesiólogo*

Hospital

Notes / *Notas*

Name

Date

Doctor(s)

Anesthesiologist

Hospital

Notes

Name

Date

Doctor(s)

Anesthesiologist

Hospital

Notes

Name

Date

Doctor(s)

Anesthesiologist

Hospital

Notes

Name / *Nombre*

Date / *Fecha*

Doctor(s) / *Médico(s)*

Anesthesiologist / *Anestesiólogo*

Hospital

Notes / *Notas*

Name

Date

Doctor(s)

Anesthesiologist

Hospital

Notes

Name

Date

Doctor(s)

Anesthesiologist

Hospital

Notes

Name

Date

Doctor(s)

Anesthesiologist

Hospital

Notes

Transfusions

Type / *Tipo*	Date / *Fecha*
Location / *Lugar*	
Reactions / *Reacciones*	

Type	Date
Location	
Reactions	

Type	Date
Location	
Reactions	

Type	Date
Location	
Reactions	

Type	Date
Location	
Reactions	

Type	Date
Location	
Reactions	

Type / *Tipo*	Date / *Fecha*
Location / *Lugar*	
Reactions / *Reacciones*	

Type	Date
Location	
Reactions	

Type	Date
Location	
Reactions	

Type	Date
Location	
Reactions	

Type	Date
Location	
Reactions	

Type	Date
Location	
Reactions	

Transfusions

Type / *Tipo*	Date / *Fecha*
Location / *Lugar*	
Reactions / *Reacciones*	

Type	Date
Location	
Reactions	

Type	Date
Location	
Reactions	

Type	Date
Location	
Reactions	

Type	Date
Location	
Reactions	

Type	Date
Location	
Reactions	

Type / *Tipo*	Date / *Fecha*
Location / *Lugar*	
Reactions / *Reacciones*	

Type	Date
Location	
Reactions	

Type	Date
Location	
Reactions	

Type	Date
Location	
Reactions	

Type	Date
Location	
Reactions	

Type	Date
Location	
Reactions	

Chemotherapy

Location / *Lugar*	Date(s) / *Fecha*

Comments / *Comentarios*

Location	Date(s)

Comments

Location	Date(s)

Comments

Location	Date(s)

Comments

Location	Date(s)

Comments

Location	Date(s)

Comments

Location	Date(s)

Comments

Location	Date(s)

Comments

Location / *Lugar*	Date(s) / *Fecha*
Comments / *Comentarios*	

Location	Date(s)
Comments	

Location	Date(s)
Comments	

Location	Date(s)
Comments	

Location	Date(s)
Comments	

Location	Date(s)
Comments	

Location	Date(s)
Comments	

Location	Date(s)
Comments	

Chemotherapy

Location / *Lugar*	Date(s) / *Fecha*

Comments / *Comentarios*

Location	Date(s)

Comments

Location	Date(s)

Comments

Location	Date(s)

Comments

Location	Date(s)

Comments

Location	Date(s)

Comments

Location	Date(s)

Comments

Location	Date(s)

Comments

Location / *Lugar*	Date(s) / *Fecha*
Comments / *Comentarios*	

Location	Date(s)
Comments	

Location	Date(s)
Comments	

Location	Date(s)
Comments	

Location	Date(s)
Comments	

Location	Date(s)
Comments	

Location	Date(s)
Comments	

Location	Date(s)
Comments	

Chemotherapy

Location / *Lugar*	Date(s) / *Fecha*
Comments / *Comentarios*	

Location	Date(s)
Comments	

Location	Date(s)
Comments	

Location	Date(s)
Comments	

Location	Date(s)
Comments	

Location	Date(s)
Comments	

Location	Date(s)
Comments	

Location	Date(s)
Comments	

Location / *Lugar*	Date(s) / *Fecha*
Comments / *Comentarios*	

Location	Date(s)
Comments	

Location	Date(s)
Comments	

Location	Date(s)
Comments	

Location	Date(s)
Comments	

Location	Date(s)
Comments	

Location	Date(s)
Comments	

Location	Date(s)
Comments	

Transplants

Type / *Tipo*

Date / *Fecha*

Hospital

Doctor(s) / *Médico(s)*

Notes / *Notas*

Type

Date

Hospital

Doctor(s)

Notes

Type

Date

Hospital

Doctor(s)

Notes

Type

Date

Hospital

Doctor(s)

Notes

Type

Date

Hospital

Doctor(s)

Notes

Type / *Tipo*

Date / *Fecha*

Hospital

Doctor(s) / *Médico(s)*

Notes / *Notas*

Type

Date

Hospital

Doctor(s)

Notes

Type

Date

Hospital

Doctor(s)

Notes

Type

Date

Hospital

Doctor(s)

Notes

Type

Date

Hospital

Doctor(s)

Notes

Other Procedures

Type / *Tipo*	
Date / *Fecha*	
Hospital	
Doctor(s) / *Médico(s)*	
Notes / *Notas*	
Type	
Date	
Hospital	
Doctor(s)	
Notes	
Type	
Date	
Hospital	
Doctor(s)	
Notes	
Type	
Date	
Hospital	
Doctor(s)	
Notes	
Type	
Date	
Hospital	
Doctor(s)	
Notes	

Type / *Tipo*

Date / *Fecha*

Hospital

Doctor(s) / *Médico(s)*

Notes / *Notas*

Type

Date

Hospital

Doctor(s)

Notes

Type

Date

Hospital

Doctor(s)

Notes

Type

Date

Hospital

Doctor(s)

Notes

Type

Date

Hospital

Doctor(s)

Notes

Other Procedures

Type / *Tipo*

Date / *Fecha*

Hospital

Doctor(s) / *Médico(s)*

Notes / *Notas*

Type

Date

Hospital

Doctor(s)

Notes

Type

Date

Hospital

Doctor(s)

Notes

Type

Date

Hospital

Doctor(s)

Notes

Type

Date

Hospital

Doctor(s)

Notes

Type / *Tipo*

Date / *Fecha*

Hospital

Doctor(s) / *Médico(s)*

Notes / *Notas*

Type

Date

Hospital

Doctor(s)

Notes

Type

Date

Hospital

Doctor(s)

Notes

Type

Date

Hospital

Doctor(s)

Notes

Type

Date

Hospital

Doctor(s)

Notes

Other Procedures

Type / *Tipo*

Date / *Fecha*

Hospital

Doctor(s) / *Médico(s)*

Notes / *Notas*

Type

Date

Hospital

Doctor(s)

Notes

Type

Date

Hospital

Doctor(s)

Notes

Type

Date

Hospital

Doctor(s)

Notes

Type

Date

Hospital

Doctor(s)

Notes

Type / *Tipo*

Date / *Fecha*

Hospital

Doctor(s) / *Médico(s)*

Notes / *Notas*

Type

Date

Hospital

Doctor(s)

Notes

Type

Date

Hospital

Doctor(s)

Notes

Type

Date

Hospital

Doctor(s)

Notes

Type

Date

Hospital

Doctor(s)

Notes

Other Procedures

Type / *Tipo*
Date / *Fecha*
Hospital
Doctor(s) / *Médico(s)*
Notes / *Notas*
Type
Date
Hospital
Doctor(s)
Notes
Type
Date
Hospital
Doctor(s)
Notes
Type
Date
Hospital
Doctor(s)
Notes
Type
Date
Hospital
Doctor(s)
Notes

Type / *Tipo*

Date / *Fecha*

Hospital

Doctor(s) / *Médico(s)*

Notes / *Notas*

Type

Date

Hospital

Doctor(s)

Notes

Type

Date

Hospital

Doctor(s)

Notes

Type

Date

Hospital

Doctor(s)

Notes

Type

Date

Hospital

Doctor(s)

Notes

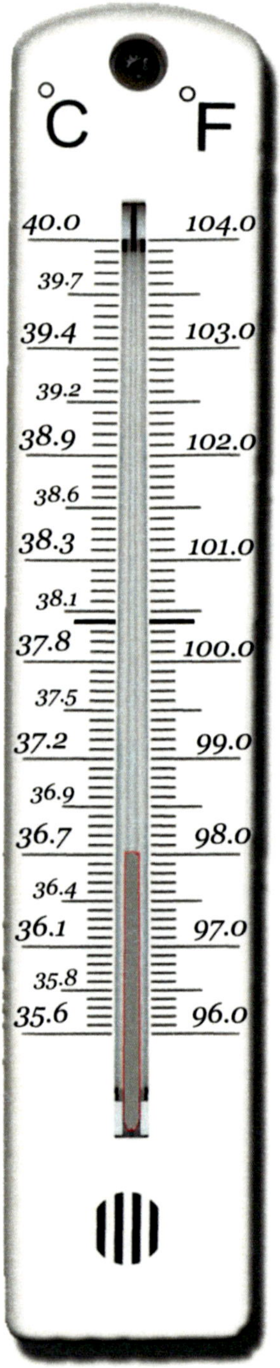

Temperature Conversion

Celsius	Fahrenheit
36.0	96.8
36.1	**97.0**
36.2	97.2
36.3	97.4
36.4	97.6
36.6	97.8
36.7	**98.0**
36.8	98.2
36.9	98.4
37.0	98.6
37.1	98.8
37.2	**99.0**
37.3	99.2
37.4	99.4
37.6	99.6
37.7	99.8
37.8	**100.0**
37.9	100.2
38.0	100.4
38.1	100.6
38.2	100.8
38.3	**101.0**
38.4	101.2
38.6	101.4
38.7	101.6
38.8	101.8
38.9	**102.0**
39.0	102.2
39.1	102.4
39.2	102.6
39.3	102.8
39.4	**103.0**
39.6	103.2
39.7	103.4
39.8	103.6
39.9	103.8
40.0	**104.0**

Temperatura

date/time	temp	date/time	temp

Temperature

date/time	temp	date/time	temp

Temperatura

date/time	temp	date/time	temp

Temperature

date/time	temp	date/time	temp

Temperatura

date/time	temp	date/time	temp

Notes / Phone Numbers

Notes / Phone Numbers

Notas / Numeros de Teléfono

Notes / Phone Numbers

Notas / Numeros de Teléfono

Notes / Phone Numbers

January / Enero

S	M	T	W	T	F	S

February / Febrero

S	M	T	W	T	F	S

March / Marzo

S	M	T	W	T	F	S

April / Abril

S	M	T	W	T	F	S

May / Mayo

S	M	T	W	T	F	S

June /Junio

S	M	T	W	T	F	S

July / Julio

S	M	T	W	T	F	S

August / Agosto

S	M	T	W	T	F	S

September / Septiembre

S	M	T	W	T	F	S

October / Octubre

S	M	T	W	T	F	S

November / Noviembre

S	M	T	W	T	F	S

December / Diciembre

S	M	T	W	T	F	S

Appendix B: General Chart

Appendix C: Weekly Sugar Graph

Date	Sunday		Monday		Tuesday		Wednesday		Thursday		Friday		Saturday	
Sugar	AM	PM	AM	PM	AM	PM	AM	PM	AM	PM	AM	PM	AM	PM
>225														
201-225														
176-200														
151-175														
126-150														
100-125														
75-100														
50-75														
25-50														
0-25														

Date	Sunday		Monday		Tuesday		Wednesday		Thursday		Friday		Saturday	
Sugar	AM	PM	AM	PM	AM	PM	AM	PM	AM	PM	AM	PM	AM	PM
>225														
201-225														
176-200														
151-175														
126-150														
100-125														
75-100														
50-75														
25-50														
0-25														

Appendix D: Six Months Chart

	Sunday		Monday		Tuesday		Wednesday		Thursday		Friday		Saturday	
	AM	PM	AM	PM	AM	PM	AM	PM	AM	PM	AM	PM	AM	PM

	Sunday		Monday		Tuesday		Wednesday		Thursday		Friday		Saturday	
	AM	PM	AM	PM	AM	PM	AM	PM	AM	PM	AM	PM	AM	PM

CDC Centers for Disease Control and Prevention
Your Online Source for Credible Health Information

http://www.cdc.gov/

FamilyDoctor.org
health information for the whole family

healthfinder.gov
Your Source for Reliable Health Information

HIV InSite

http://hivinsite.ucsf.edu/InSite

KidsHealth.org®

MAYO CLINIC

http://www.mayoclinic.com/

NOAH New York Online Access to Health
Acceso Computerizado de la Salud en Nueva York

http://www.noah-health.org/

NATIONAL CANCER INSTITUTE

http://www.cancer.gov/

American Cancer Society

http://www.cancer.org/

Medem

Connecting Physicians and Patients

http://www.medem.com/

Families of Children with Cancer

http://www.fcco.org/

WebMD

Better information. Better health.

http://www.webmd.com/

American Diabetes Association.

Cure • Care • Commitment.

http://www.diabetes.org/

U.S. Department of Health & Human Services

HHS.gov

American Heart Association®

Learn and Live℠

http://www.americanheart.org/

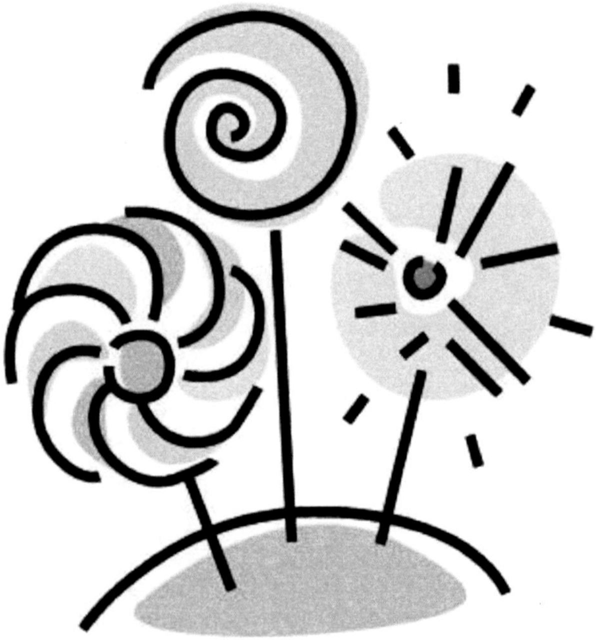

Printed in the U.S.A.

9 780977 723522